NEWI

To renew books ring the Helpdesk
01978 293237

Depression in Elderly People

Simon Lovestone MRCPsych
Senior Lecturer in Old Age Psychiatry

Robert Howard MRCPsych
Senior Lecturer in Old Age Psychiatry

Section of Old Age Psychiatry
Institute of Psychiatry
London, UK

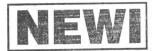

MARTIN DUNITZ

First published in the United Kingdom
in 1996 by

Martin Dunitz Ltd
The Livery House
7–9 Pratt Street
London NW1 0AE

A CIP record for this book is available from the
British Library.

ISBN 1-85317-245-6

Printed and bound in Spain by Cayfosa

Contents

Foreword

Depression in the elderly is an underdiagnosed and under-treated disorder. If all forms of depression are included, the prevalence is as high as 15% in people over 65 years of age. There is a large heterogeneity in both aetiology and response to treatment of depression in the elderly compared with younger people, and the cause is often multifactorial. Because it has an atypical symptomatology and there is insufficient information about the disorder, patients and their relatives are not always aware that depression is present. The symptoms are instead regarded as part of normal ageing by local social services and general practitioners.

Today, treatment is available for depression in elderly people. If local social services provide a good social network, modern psychopharmacology (e.g. selective serotonin re-uptake inhibitors) is applied and cognitive therapy, or possibly electroconvulsive therapy, is used in patients who do not respond to drug treatment alone, then depression in the elderly can be treated successfully.

An important task is to spread information about depression in the elderly to the staff in outpatient services. In this book, Simon Lovestone and Robert Howard present such information in a comprehensive, easily understandable way. Valuable advice is given for identification, diagnosis and treatment of the disorder. The book can be recommended for general practitioners and other workers in the front line of medical care. It is of great use also to specialists who meet elderly people in their practice.

Carl Gerhard Gottfries MD PhD
Professor of Psychiatry
Institute of Neuroscience
Göteborg University, Sweden

Introduction

It is perhaps not surprising that elderly people become depressed. The final decades of life bring with them a shrinking social world, increasing ill health and reduced social standing. Whether because depression in the elderly is superficially understandable or because older people are reluctant to seek help, depression in the elderly has, in the past, been under-diagnosed and is often now under-treated. This is the unacceptable face of ageism; underlying this book is our experience that the elderly can, and should, remain free from depressive illness.

Epidemiology and classification of depression

Rates of depression in the community

The measured rates of depression in the elderly (both prevalence and incidence) depend both upon populations studied and on definitions of depression used (Fig. 1). Community-based studies find symptoms of depression in up to 15% of the elderly; the prevalence of major depressive disorders is lower (<4%). Rates of major depressive illness do not show a marked gender difference, although symptoms of depression are considerably more common in women. Epidemiology has failed to fully resolve the issue as to whether the incidence of depressive illness rises in the elderly. Although a substantial number of the elderly have significant symptoms of depression at any time, the prevalence of major depressive disorder is broadly similar to that in the younger population. For example, using the Geriatric Mental State (a widely-used research instrument in this population) in a large study of over 65 year-olds in Britain, the prevalence of major depressive disorder was found to be 2–4% and the prevalence of minor depression to be 11% for women and 5% for men. One of the world's largest population based studies – the Epidemiologic Catchment Area (ECA) Study – found a prevalence of major depressive illness in the community-dwelling elderly of only 1%. Other studies suggest that the very elderly may be relatively resistant to depressive illnesses.

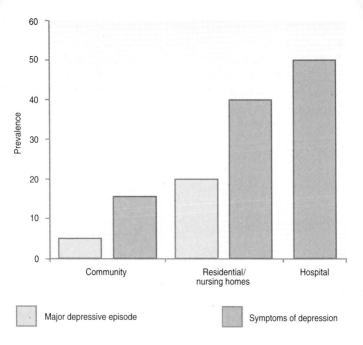

Figure 1
Rates of depression in the elderly.

Depression in other settings

The low rates of depressive illness reported in the ECA study may reflect the community setting of this research. Such studies cannot be extrapolated to all populations of old people. Depression is relatively more common in elderly general practice attenders and is present in a very substantial proportion of hospitalized elderly and residents in nursing homes. A series of studies has found a prevalence of major depressive illness of approximately 20% in nursing home residents with up to 40% of residents in both nursing homes and local authority residential homes showing some signs and symptoms of depression (Fig. 1). Measuring rates of depression in the hospitalized elderly is difficult because of co-existing serious physical illness, yet some studies show that nearly half of all such patients have some signs of depression.

The reason for the discrepancy between prevalence of depression in the community and in residential settings is not entirely clear. To some extent the elderly living in the community represent a healthy survivor population, and those in residential and nursing homes represent a population selected for increased physical morbidity and psychiatric vulnerability. In other words depression may have been one of the causes for a move to a residential care setting. However, it might be that the increased prevalence of depression in elderly people in residential care settings is also to some extent a consequence of leaving independent dwelling in the community. The move to residential and nursing home care brings with it loss of independence and loss of privacy. The family house, perhaps a lifelong home, is relinquished and the elderly person has to become accustomed to life in a communal setting – a situation usually encountered only in boarding schools or the armed forces. Given these loss events and the increased vulnerability of older people in care settings, the increased prevalence of depression should be predicted and appropriate measures taken to address this need. The model of service provision to this group of elderly will depend to a large extent upon local circumstances, but might be provided through regular outreach clinics by an old age psychiatry service, through close liaison between a community nurse and the home, or directly through the primary care team providing a comprehensive medical service to the home.

Symptoms of depression, then, are common in the elderly and significant depressive illness constitutes a substantial burden to individuals and to their relatives. Depressive illness is present in between a quarter and a half of those elderly patients in hospital and in residential homes. These individuals suffer substantial morbidity and constitute a major clinical and economic burden to health and social services.

Suicide in the elderly

Depression causes not only morbidity but also mortality, and prevention of suicide is a major treatment goal of the old age psychiatrist. The elderly are, if anything, more vulnerable to suicide than younger depressives and a quarter of all UK suicides are in those aged over 65 years. The suicide rate for men rises steadily with age and in many Western countries accelerates in the very elderly. This trend may be changing with a somewhat reduced acceleration in the elderly. Rates for women are lower than for men at all ages and women show a plateau and even reduction in rates in the elderly (Fig. 2). However, despite this and despite some differences between countries, late life suicide is a major health concern.

Foremost among risk factors for suicide are loneliness and social isolation. Bereavement is a major cause of isolation in the elderly and there is some evidence that the newly bereaved are particularly vulnerable. In younger age groups suicide shows an association with social class, being more common in those in the higher social classes. In the elderly this situation is partially reversed. Alcohol is a risk factor at all ages although alcohol abuse in the elderly may go unnoticed.

The pattern of an elderly man, living alone and recently bereaved, suffering from depression and possibly drinking

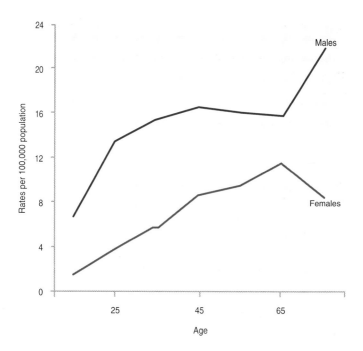

Figure 2
Suicide rates in England and Wales 1982–1984.

more alcohol should indicate to the clinician the need to pay close attention to suicidal intention. It is a dangerous myth that those who talk about killing themselves rarely do so – many if not most successful suicides have consulted a general practitioner, for example, in the very recent past. There can be a reluctance to interrogate the elderly about suicide, not least because interviewers are invariably from a younger generation. However, assessment of suicide risk in the depressed elderly and those with chronic physical illness is a critical task.

Nomenclature

Psychiatry has suffered from a preoccupation with the classification of affective disorders over recent years. Two major diagnostic systems are currently in use and are summarized in Table 1. In clinical practice, however, a number of syndromes predominate:

- Major depressive illness equates broadly to that category previously known as psychotic or endogenous depression.

- Minor depressive illness was previously subsumed under the unfortunate rubric *neurotic depression*, and is frequently present as an admixture with anxiety.

- The third type of illness occasionally encountered in the elderly is chronic dysthymia – the state of 'always having been depressed'. This is relatively less common in the elderly although young depressives do grow old with their depression – the graduate depressive illness. Whether these cases are best treated by specialists in psychiatry for the elderly is a point of some contention. Where there are age-specific features – such as frailty, physical illness, disability or even great age – then specialist intervention is indicated.

- Finally, depression can occur secondary to physical illness, including dementia.

The clinical presentation of these common syndromes will be discussed in the chapter starting on page 21.

ICD-10

- Depressive episode
  - severe
  - moderate
  - mild
  - other/unspecified

- Bipolar affective disorder

- Recurrent depressive disorders

- Persistent mood (affective) states (including dysthmyia)

- Other disorders of mood

DSM-IV

• Depressive disorders	Major depressive disorder Dysthymic disorders Depressive disorder not otherwise specified
• Bipolar disorders	Bipolar I disorder (mania usually with depression) Bipolar II disorder (depression with hypomania) Cyclothymic disorder Bipolar disorder not otherwise specified
• Mood disorder due to a general medical condition	
• Substance-induced mood disorder	
• Other disorders of mood	

Table 1
ICD-10 and DSM-IV classifications of depression.

Aetiology

The elderly are exposed to many putative risk factors for depression. Increased physical ill health, psychosocial factors and an ageing brain all contribute to the high prevalence of depression in the elderly (Table 2).

Table 2
Aetiology of depression in the elderly.

Social
• Reduced social networks
• Loneliness
• Bereavement
• Poverty
• Physical ill health

Psychological

- Poor self-esteem

- Lack of capacity for intimacy

- Physical ill health

Biological

- Neuronal loss/neurotransmitter loss

- Genetic risk

- Physical ill health

Physical ill health

Indirect influence of ill health on mood

Ill health causes depressive morbidity directly and indirectly. Murphy's seminal studies demonstrated that physical ill health is a major cause of vulnerability to depression. New physical ill health events frequently precipitate depressive episodes and also contribute to chronicity. Chronic illness in the elderly also contributes to depression indirectly through restriction of mobility, increased dependence on others and by causing chronic pain or discomfort. Clinical experience suggests that it is not the 'medical seriousness' or threat to life itself that is so damaging to the mental health of the elderly – instead it is those aspects of physical illness that result in loss events that correlate most closely with depressed mood. Loss events in the elderly are not only the somewhat obvious and universal losses of retirement and bereavement but also more fundamental losses of dignity and a role in life. Physical illness commonly results in the loss of mobility and the loss of ability to care fully for oneself. Accompanying this are the fears of increasing ill health, the fear of falling and the fear of becoming a burden.

Loss of sleep and chronic pain are frequent precipitants of depression. In addition relatively less common symptoms such as tinnitus or pruritus can become dominant in the elderly and cause seemingly intractable and serious depressive episodes. The interaction between ill health and depressive mood is complex and bidirectional. Just as chronic ill health contributes to a poor prognosis of depression, so too can depression point to a poor prognosis of physical illness. One UK prospective study has demonstrated a higher mortality in depressed, physically ill inpatients than in the non-depressed inpatients.

Direct influence of ill health on mood

In addition to an indirect influence of ill health on mood, some disorders cause depression by more direct mechanisms (Fig. 3). Stroke is associated with a high incidence of major depression (20–24% in recent studies), particularly in the elderly. Depression is more common in those with larger lesions and more pronounced functional disability. Despite early enthusiasm, depression has not been consistently associated with a particular anatomical location of stroke.

Other neurological disorders are associated with depression. Many patients with Parkinson's disease appear depressed, although whether the rates of depression are substantially higher than for other illnesses accompanied by chronic disability is unclear. Depression precedes motor signs in many cases

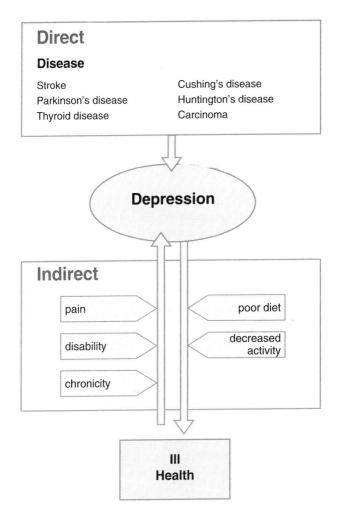

Figure 3
Interactions between physical health and mood.

of Huntington's disease and, although the onset is most commonly in mid-life, direct molecular diagnosis following the discovery of the Huntington's disease gene mutation has enabled the recognition of significant numbers of the elderly with this condition. First presentation of carcinoma (particularly lung and brain) can be as depression, and thyroid and steroid abnormalities are important, if rare, direct physical causes of altered mood.

Drugs

The elderly are particularly prone to being the recipients of, and indeed the sufferers from, polypharmacy (Fig. 4). A wide range of class of drugs are associated with depressive mood, although it has to be said that the mechanism whereby some classes of drugs appear to affect mood are unknown (Table 3). Polypharmacy is widely accepted as bad practice in the elderly and leads to an increased frequency of side-effects, drug interactions and poor compliance in addition to the effects on mood. However, preventing polypharmacy can be difficult, particularly given the multiple pathologies that may be encountered in an individual. All those who treat the elderly should strive to keep prescribing to a minimum and to ensure ongoing review of all medications (Fig. 4). Periodic medical interventions such as hospital admission or over 75s checks by general practitioners can be useful occasions to check medications and cease prescribing all but essential drugs.

Neurobiological factors

It is a point of considerable interest and contention as to whether the ageing brain itself is more vulnerable to depression. Jacoby and Levy demonstrated by computed tomography (CT) that cortical tissue density in a depressed group of patients was more similar to a group of demented patients than to normal controls. Functional evidence of reduced cor-

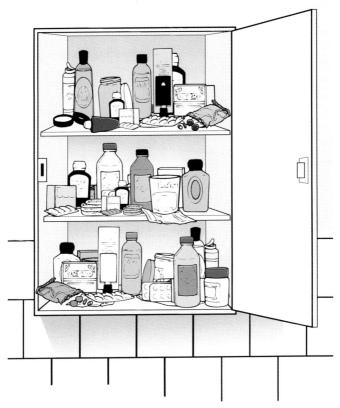

Figure 4
Polypharmacy in the elderly is both common and dangerous.

tical reserve comes from evidence that cognitive impairments are present during depressive episodes and fail to restore to normal after recovery of mood in a substantial proportion of patients. These studies suggest that depression in

- Digoxin

- L-Dopa

- Steroids

- Beta-blockers

- Other antihypertensives

- Chronic benzodiazepine prescription

- Phenobarbitone

- Neuroleptics in chronic use

Table 3
Drugs causing depression.

the elderly can result from a neurodegenerative process just as depression can be a symptom of dementia. While a genetic susceptibility to depression has been widely recognized, such an association is far less robust in the elderly.

Monoaminergic function has been implicated in depressive illness for many decades. The first wave of antidepressants increase aminergic function, by reducing reuptake by blocking presynaptic receptors (tricyclic antidepressants) or by reducing breakdown in the synaptic cleft (monoamine oxidase inhibitors). These compounds are very effective but are not specific and affect both the noradrenergic and serotonergic systems. Compounds specific to each of these neurotransmitters have been developed and are extremely effective in treating depression. Serotonin function has been implicated in both suicide and depression by direct measurement of metabolites in cerebrospinal fluid and in the brain. However, relatively few studies have attempted to identify functional brain deficits particularly relevant in the elderly. Evidence does exist that there is an age-dependent reduction in activity of noradrenergic, serotonergic and dopaminergic markers in the brain. For serotonergic function in particular, the activity is reduced by half in 80-year-olds when compared to 60-year-olds.

Neuroendocrinological changes have also been suggested as factors modifying vulnerability to depression, and control of hormonal regulation may be impaired in the elderly. Despite a large body of research, neurotransmitter and neuroendocrinological studies to date have shed a little light, but very little enlightenment, on the causes of depression in any age group.

Psychosocial factors

Personality
Some authors have suggested that depressed patients with an onset of illness in later life tend to have more robust personalities than the younger depressed. Those late onset depressives who present with predominantly neurotic symptoms have often been anxiety prone premorbidly. The relationship between personality and depression is a difficult issue and one that is far from understood. However, the elderly with a first episode of depression in late life have long had a fully formed personality and a life experience behind them and this can aid recovery, in contrast to some people who experience an onset of depression in early life.

Social supports

Specific vulnerability factors for the development of depression in young patients include loss of mother before the age of 11 and lack of a relationship with a confidante or intimate. While the first of these factors has not been confirmed in all studies of elderly depressed patients, the lifelong lack of a capacity for intimacy may be important and some studies have suggested that, particularly for men, the absence of a current confidante is the most important vulnerability factor in the development of depression.

Being married is a protective factor against depression, especially for men. Depressive episodes are more common in the widowed or the divorced although this does not simply result from the absence of a partner as those who have never married have relatively low rates of depression.

Caring for another elderly person is, however, associated with depression even when that person is a spouse. Prevalence of depression in spouse carers of partners with Alzheimer's disease have been reported in some studies to be as high as 50%, although other studies report lower rates. Caring for a spouse with dementia always carries some degree of burden although this burden does not always translate to depression as an outcome. Many aspects of caring can be positive and life enhancing especially when given to a loved spouse. Depression as an outcome is more common when the carer looks after a spouse with behavioural disturbance – such as wandering or aggression. We have studied spouses of patients with depression and find no increase in depressive episodes in these carers in contrast to the carers of those patients with dementia.

As increasing numbers of couples become old together and as services for the mentally frail become increasingly focused on care in the community, it is to be expected that depression in elderly carers will be an increasing problem.

Life events

Severe life events are more common in depressed patients during the year preceding illness development than among the healthy elderly. Examples of such events are:

- Death of a partner
- Major financial problems
- Enforced removal from home

Since so many elderly people will suffer such adverse life events it is tempting to ask why more of them do not become depressed. Making a distinction between a depressive illness requiring drug treatment and the low mood accompanying a bereavement is often difficult.

Death of a partner has been suggested to have more impact on an elderly person if it was unexpected. However, studies have not confirmed this finding and the death of the spouse after a long illness can be equally traumatic. The weeks immediately following a bereavement are a period of high risk for depressive episodes with the recently bereaved requiring additional support. Anniversaries of bereavements can also be traumatic and some fine old age psychiatry services make a point of visiting patients with a history of depression at or around this time.

We know of little research in this area, but clinical experience suggests that the death or severe illness of a child is an appalling event for the elderly and can initiate major depressive episodes. Parents of severely disabled children often worry about their future and this becomes of more acute concern as the children become adults and as the parent reaches an advanced age. We have encountered major depression in parents of patients with schizophrenia with these elderly people voicing concerns for the child's well-being in years to come.

Finally, severe adverse life events and trauma can induce a syndrome of anxiety and depression with many of the features of post-traumatic stress disorder (PTSD). Anniversaries of long distant traumatic events can also induce such syndromes, and anxiety and depression occurring at the time of and indeed apparently related to the 50th anniversary celebrations of the end of World War II have been reported.

Clinical presentation of depression in the elderly

The entire range of clinical symptoms of early onset depression also occurs in the elderly. Historical notions of a unique presentation of late life depression – the hypochondriacal depressive or the neurovegetative depressive – are largely discounted today. However, recognizing depression in the elderly can require special skills and experience. In particular, differentiating the psychological sequelae of physical disorder from depressive illness, and the somatic symptoms of depression from the effects of systemic disease can be difficult. The particular challenge for old age psychiatry is that all can occur together in a single individual (Table 4).

The elderly person with depression may complain of low mood but often presents with loss of energy, loss of enjoyment, sleeplessness or aches and pains. Assessing reduced energy requires a different approach in the elderly as a reduction in energy accompanying old age is almost invariable. A recent change or a constant feeling of exhaustion or inertia, even at rest, are useful pointers. Loss of enjoyment, or anhedonia, in the elderly is not normal, despite the prejudices of the young. In assessing anhedonia in the elderly it is helpful to identify first those aspects of life that normally give enjoyment to the patient. Ask about enjoyment of television or visits from the family, for instance. Enjoyment of the company of younger members of the family, grandchildren or great grandchildren, is very rarely lost in the elderly except in the context of depression.

Table 4
Diagnosis of depression, adapted from ICD-10 and DSM IV.

ICD-10

Common symptoms of depression
- Depressed mood
- Loss of interest
- Loss of energy

Other symptoms of depression
- Reduced concentration
- Reduced self esteem
- Guilt feelings
- Pessimism regarding the future
- Self harm or suicidal ideas
- Altered sleep
- Decreased appetite

Mild depression
- At least two common and two other symptoms
- Patient may be distressed but can function well

Moderate depression
- At least two common and three or four other symptoms
- Duration is at least two weeks and function is impaired

Severe depression
- All three common and at least four other symptoms
- Symptoms are severe in intensity and function is profoundly affected

DSM-IV (Major Depression)

Five or more of the following symptoms have been present during the same two week period nearly every day. At least one of the symptoms is either (1) depressed mood or (2) loss of interest or pleasure.

- Depressed mood most of the day
- Markedly diminished interest or pleasure in normal activities
- Significant weight loss or weight gain
- Insomnia or hypersomnia
- Psychomotor agitation or retardation
- Fatigue or loss of energy
- Feelings of worthlessness or excessive guilt
- Reduced ability to concentrate
- Recurrent thoughts of death, suicidal thoughts or attempts

There must be clinically significant distress or impairment in functioning. The symptoms must not be due to the effects of a general medical condition or to the effects of a substance (e.g. drug abuse or medication)

Sleeplessness is a difficult area to assess and is often a problem for the non-depressed elderly (Table 5). Particular patterns of sleep loss such as early morning waking are useful pointers, as are depressive thought contents or ruminations when awake at night. The elderly require less sleep and can be woken by, for example, nocturia. It is therefore important to enquire about the behaviour of the patient when they awake in the night. Appropriate management of insomnia in the elderly requires attention to sleep hygiene (adjusting the timing of meals, making the bedroom a place for sleep only and preventing daytime naps) before pharmacological management.

Causes

- Nocturia
- Reduced need for sleep
- Day time napping
- Alcohol
- Depression and anxiety
- Excessive worry about sleep pattern
- Nocturnal confusion

Assessments

- Informant history – not always available
- Assess energy and activity by day
- Physical examination and subsequent investigations
- Mental state
- Assess expected sleep pattern
- Sleep chart

Management

- Information – the elderly expect more sleep than they need
- Sleep only at night
- Increase activity by day
- Keep the bedroom as a place for sleep only
- Reduce alcohol intake
- Adjust meal times (major meal early in evening)
- Hypnotics rarely useful in long term management

Table 5
Insomnia in the elderly.

Presentation with physical symptoms requires close attention to the pattern of the symptomatology as well as a systematic search for non-disclosed symptoms of depression. Co-morbidity is common and often investigation and treatment of both depression and physical illness are necessary simultaneously.

Deteriorating self care, a change in eating habit or loss of weight can all be the earliest indications of depression, but may also be the presenting signs of a dementia. Cognitive assessment of the elderly depressed should never be omitted. Simple tests of memory include the abbreviated mental test score and the somewhat longer mini mental state examination. Cognitive impairment in the depressed can indicate a dementia although it may be secondary to depressed mood. However, if the cognitive impairment is secondary, then an improvement to some degree should be observed with treatment. A persistently impaired cognition does not in any way preclude treatment of the depressive symptomatology, but does indicate that further assessment will be necessary. In addition to prompting an investigation of the cognitive impairment, an assessment of the patient's functional ability and an occupational therapy assessment of the home might be indicated. Should the cognitive impairment prove to be due to dementia then an appropriate management plan will include attention to home care facilities and discussions with relatives about the most appropriate place of residence to meet the needs of the patient.

Finally, psychotic symptoms and severe depression in the elderly can be dramatic. Delusions of guilt or poverty or delusions that internal organs are rotten, diseased or absent are all classically described, but are in fact rarely encountered outside hospitals. Auditory hallucinations of a derogatory nature and somatic hallucinations also occur, although visual hallucinations should suggest the search for another diagnosis.

Syndromes of depression in the elderly

Most episodes of depression can be described well enough for clinical practice as minor or major depressive illness. However, a number of other syndromic presentations occur in the elderly.

Agitated depression

Increased activity, relentless pacing, incessant hand wringing can all point to a picture of agitated depression. This presentation is particularly difficult for relatives, and the elderly spouse of a person with agitated depression and insomnia should be drawn aside and assessed in their own right. The spouse will, not infrequently, be found to be exhausted and to be suffering from some aspects of depression themselves. The management of the elderly agitated depressed patient (and indeed other syndromes of depression) will include consideration of measures designed to support the spouse such as day respite care.

Anxiety and depression

Both somatic and psychic symptoms of anxiety co-exist with depression and anxiety can frequently dominate the clinical picture (Table 6). Increased generalized anxiety as well as phobic states occur together with depression and studies suggest that anxiety is 15 to 20 times more common in elderly subjects with depression. Physical illness is associated with anxiety in the elderly and, as with depression, the relationship is complex. Anxiety can cause physical symptoms that can easily be mistaken for physical illness and severe anxiety can cause exhaustion and dehydration. Physical illness that threatens life or loss of independence can frequently be a source and cause of anxiety.

Masked depression

Absence of the usual appearance of low mood should not preclude a diagnosis of depression. Whether because of a wish to avoid becoming a burden or because of the determination of the current cohort of the elderly to 'put a brave face upon it', late life depression can be masked by a smiling visage. 'Masked depression' is a rather old-fashioned term but does seem to apply to a particular group of older people with depression. This does not prevent the experienced from searching for other signs and symptoms of depression.

Psychological	Physical
• Worrying	• Restlessness
• Fearfulness	• Breathlessness and hyperventilation
• Apprehension	• Sweating
• Increased vigilance	• Headaches and muscular pains
• Poor concentration and memory	• Stomach cramps
	• Vomiting and diarrhoea
	• Palpitations

Table 6
Anxiety symptoms in the elderly.

Pseudodementia

Pseudodementia is a term that has been used to describe many different presentations. The most common use of the term is for the patient with depression who presents with apparent loss of memory. In contrast to the demented, however, the depressive pseudodementia patient is unwilling to attempt cognitive assessment, is able precisely to date the onset of this impairment and is acutely aware that memory is deficient. Other symptoms and signs of depression are usually present and diagnostic confusion is often the result of an overassiduous dependence on the cognitive assessment (in contrast to the history) to diagnose dementia.

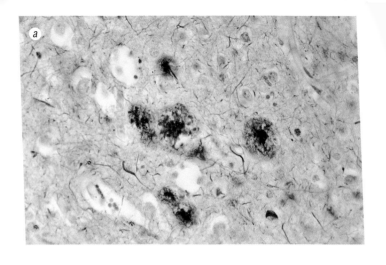

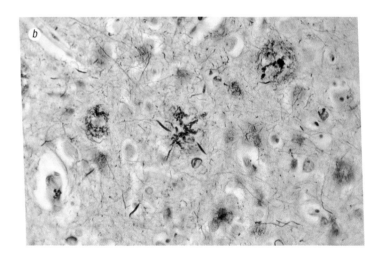

Figure 5 (a and b)
Neuritic plaques containing amyloid as found in Alzheimer's disease.

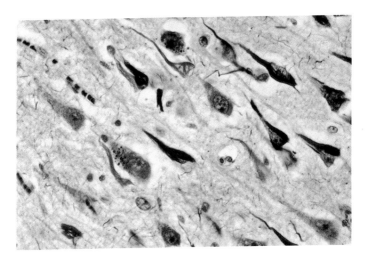

Figure 6
Neurofibrillary tangles in Alzheimer's disease.

Depression secondary to dementia

The neurodegeneration of Alzheimer's disease and other dementias results in a loss of brain tissue, as well as the characteristic neuritic plaques and neurofibrillary tangles (Figs. 5 and 6). As well as the invariable symptom of loss of memory, depression frequently occurs as a secondary symptom. Often presenting relatively early in the condition, symptoms of depression include lowered mood and tearfulness or a change in behaviour. Depression is thought to be more common in non-Alzheimer disease dementias, although rigorous studies to test this hypothesis have not yet been performed. Depression as part of a dementia syndrome can occur in the early stages, perhaps as a result of retained insight. Even partial knowledge of a deterioration and an indication of a progressive loss of ability is profoundly distressing. We recall a pair of sisters, both with dementia but one more advanced than the other, who were seriously depressed. The least demented of the two realized that her sister was seriously ill and became extremely distraught. The sister with more advanced dementia had little insight but repeated frequently that half of her brain was missing. Both sisters spent much of the day crying and increasingly refused to eat and lost considerable weight.

Depression occurring late in the course of a dementing illness might be due to loss of neurotransmitter function. In Alzheimer's disease cholinergic, noradrenergic and serotonergic function is lost. It has been hypothesized that depression and behavioural disturbance in dementia are due to reduced serotonergic function and it has been suggested that rectifying serotonergic function (with selective serotonin re-uptake inhibitors) might be useful in treating some non-cognitive symptoms in dementia, while rectifying cholinergic function is proposed to treat the cognitive deficits.

Assessment of the depressed patient

Detection of depression in the elderly by the primary health care team has undoubtedly improved over the past decade or so. However, identification is only the first step towards successful management of depression and does not always, or even often, lead to full and appropriate treatment. Nonetheless, increasing recognition of depressive illness is a major goal and should be an important component of screening the over-75s. There is no consensus as yet on procedures to screen for depression in the elderly community-dwelling population, although research in this area is proceeding. One screening instrument does, however, seem promising. The Geriatric Depression Scale (GDS) was originally described as a 30-item scale for self-completion and was then condensed to a 15-item version retaining sensitivity for identifying depression. However, when assessing total health and social care needs a 15-item questionnaire is probably too long for use in primary care as a screening instrument. It has been suggested that four items of the GDS might be used in this context by general practitioners and colleagues.

4-item scale		Score 1 point	Score 0 points
1	Are you basically satisfied with your life?	No	Yes
2	Do you feel your life is empty?	Yes	No
3	Are you afraid that something bad is going to happen to you?	Yes	No
4	Do you feel happy most of the time?	No	Yes

This four-item scale is a good starting point for assessing depression and might be usefully supplemented by a checklist of vulnerability factors:

Vulnerability factors			
1	Does the patient have a history of depression?	Yes	No
2	Is the patient socially isolated?	Yes	No
3	Does the patient suffer from chronic ill health problems?	Yes	No
4	Has there been a recent bereavement?	Yes	No

This simple screening procedure could be incorporated into over-75s checks by general practitioners and be used with ease by community nurses. Elderly people scoring more than one on the GDS-4, or more than one on the vulnerability checklist, should receive a more detailed assessment as below.

The clinical history

History taking from a depressed patient is the most important aspect of assessment and there are five main points which must be addressed in every case:

1   *Family history.*
    Is there a family history of depression or other psychiatric illness?
    Have any of the patient's relatives in fact lived as long as the patient (or did they die of other causes before the age of onset of late-life depression)?

2   *Past psychiatric illness.*
    Does the patient have a personal psychiatric history of any kind?
    Is there a history of alcohol or substance abuse or have they ever been treated before for anxiety or phobic disorders?
    If there is a personal history of depression, how was this treated and what kind of recovery was seen?
    Was the patient treated with electroconvulsive therapy and did they have any adverse reactions to this or any other form of antidepressant treatment?

3   *Personality.*
    What is the patient's personality function like when well?
    Information about this aspect of their life should be gleaned from an informant who has known the patient well for several years.

4   *Social history.*
    What is the patient's best level of functioning?
    Do they live alone, do they go out, do they have any help at home?

5   *Suicide.*
    Does the patient represent a significant suicidal risk?
    Have they made previous attempts to take their own life?
    Do they admit to suicidal preoccupations or to having made actual plans?

Physical examination

The physical assessment of depressed patients is important because depressive symptoms commonly accompany medical illness. Depression may be a symptom of an actual physical illness as, for example, in Cushing's disease or occult carcinoma of the lung, large bowel or pancreas. Alternatively, depression may emerge as a secondary reaction to disability and discomfort as, for example, in a patient with Paget's disease. In addition to a routine physical examination of the major systems, the patient should be assessed for nutritional and hydration state, since they may have been failing to maintain an adequate food or fluid intake prior to presentation.

Cognitive examination

All elderly patients with depression should undergo a brief bedside cognitive examination with, for example, an instrument like the mini mental state examination (MMSE) or the abbreviated mental test score (AMTS). Depression is a common feature of early dementia and in addition mood disorder can cause impairment of memory and concentration. The AMTS can be used as a primary screen of memory impairment in all elderly subjects in the community and the MMSE as a more comprehensive cognitive screen where depression or dementia is suspected. A reduced score on either will prompt a more complete mental state and cognitive examination and repeated assessments, which should be performed as mood is treated. Patients with depression secondary to dementia will show no improvement in cognitive function as their mood improves and may continue to show a cognitive deterioration. Patients with primary depression and secondary concentration or memory problems should show some improvement in cognitive function as their mood returns to normal. Documenting this change will be important for subsequent management.

Mental State Examination

Appearance and behaviour
Is the patient's behaviour appropriate – are they crying; do they appear depressed; is eye contact good? Look for signs of anxiety or agitation. Are there signs of poor self-care either in the patient or in their home?

Mood
Does the patient feel miserable or hopeless? Enquire about sleep, appetite, energy, concentration

Speech
Is the flow of speech normal and spontaneous?

Thoughts
Does the patient have predominantly negative thoughts about themselves, their future or their environment? Do they have over-valued ideas regarding poverty or ill health? Are their frank delusions or hallucinations consistent with a psychotic depressive episode? Examine for unusual experiences or beliefs. Make a point of re-examining the risk of suicide

Investigations

Elderly patients are extremely vulnerable to metabolic distur-bances secondary to the effects of a severe depressive illness, such as failure to maintain an adequate fluid intake. For this reason, as well as to exclude some of the medical conditions implicated above, the following represent the main investiga-tions to be considered in elderly patients presenting with depression:

Urea and electrolytes

May be altered by dehydration in the severely depressed

Metabolic upset causes restlessness, agitation and confusion

It is important to detect metabolic abnormalities before commencing pharmacotherapy

Full blood count and ESR

Chronic infections can cause depression; these are suggested by a raised white cell count or elevated ESR

Anaemia causes lassitude

B_{12} and folate

Deficiency can result from a poor diet in the chronically depressed and can lead to altered cognitive function and confusion

Thyroid function tests

Abnormalities may cause depression

Chest X-ray

Carcinoma may cause depression

Chronic chest illness or heart failure contribute directly and indirectly to depression

Additional investigations which may be helpful in particular cases include:

- Syphilis serology

- Electrocardiogram (ECG)

- Electroencephalogram (EEG)

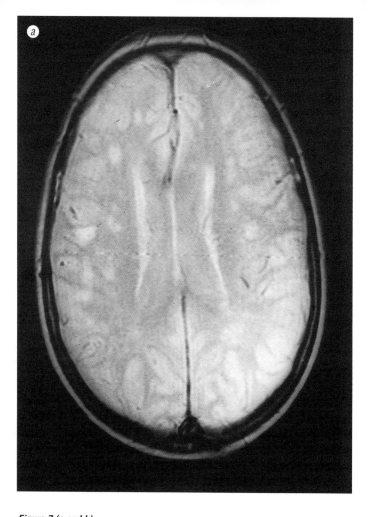

Figure 7 (a and b)
T2-weighted MRI axial images of the brain of a patient with late-life depression, showing pathological areas of signal hyperintensity around the lateral ventricles and in subcortical white matter.

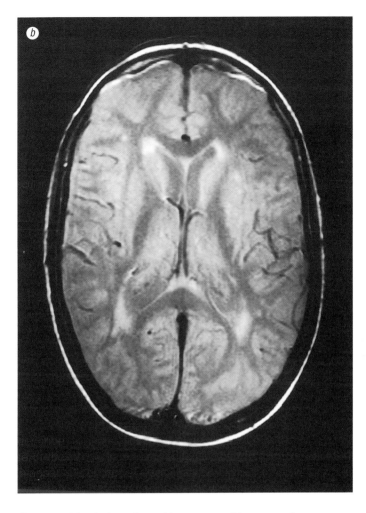

Structural brain imaging with computed tomography or magnetic resonance imaging (Fig. 7) may be helpful to demonstrate areas of cortical or subcortical cerebrovascular damage which may contribute to treatment resistance. Demonstration of gross cerebral atrophy may also indicate an associated dementia, although it is important to remember that many elderly individuals with cortical shrinkage have normal cognitive function.

Prognosis

Detection of depression in the elderly is only of value if appropriate treatment is instigated and in turn this is worthwhile only if the treatment is effective. Perhaps one reason why so many patients with depression remain under-treated in the community is the widely held view that the prognosis of depression in the elderly is particularly poor. The poor outcome of patients with late-life depression reported by Roth and his colleagues in the 1950s was apparently confirmed in the milestone papers of Murphy in the 1980s. One year after referral to an old age psychiatry service, only one-third of patients had recovered and half had a poor outcome, either relapsing or remaining depressed. Subsequent studies have, however, shed a more optimistic light on the prognosis of depression in late life with a series of studies showing over 60% recovery at one year. The interpretation of research in this area is bedevilled by subjective definitions of good or bad outcomes. Does a rapid recovery from a major depressive episode followed by an extended period of good health and active life become a bad outcome if the patient briefly relapses? While complete recovery without relapse is the goal of treatment, a brief but treatable relapse should not herald therapeutic nihilism in the elderly any more than it does in the young or middle-aged population with depression.

One undisputed poor outcome is, however, death. The mortality rate in the depressed elderly is much increased; Murphy reported that one-third of her sample had died at four year follow-up. The cause of death did not appear to be related directly to the depression itself, being mainly vascular disease or chest infection and not suicide. The reason for increased mortality in the elderly depressed is not clear. Most probably these findings result from the pattern of referral of patients to secondary care, with patients suffering from dual pathology – depression and physical illness – being referred more readily to hospital-based services.

Poor prognosis – whether for continuous illness or repeated relapse – is related to severity of illness but not to the clinical symptoms; psychotic symptoms do not seem to predict a worse outcome. By far the most important factors, however, in predicting poor outcome are those that are independently associated with the onset of depression. Physical ill health is possibly the single biggest factor, with those suffering from chronic disability or progressive illness being most vulnerable to relapse.

The outcome of depression in late life, then, is not dissimilar to the outcome of depression in younger people. The majority of patients will recover and will remain well one year later. Of those that relapse, a large proportion will have spent much of the intervening period well and active. Not surprisingly a relatively poor outcome is associated with a more severe initial episode and with chronic ill health. Treatment undoubtedly does affect prognosis – both recovery from the initial episode and maintaining subsequent remissions. Adequate initial treatment is essential and for more severe depressive episodes this may necessitate the use of electroconvulsive therapy (ECT). Indeed some of the differences in outcome in the studies on prognosis of depression in the elderly probably relate to differing use of ECT, with those centres utilising ECT demonstrating a better prognosis for their patients.

Many elderly people with depression will, however, be treated in the community by primary care teams and never reach hospital-based old age psychiatry teams. The increasing recognition of depression in the elderly by general practitioners and community nurses must be followed by adequate treatment using a combination of pharmacological and psychological approaches. The effective management of depression in the elderly calls out for a multi-disciplinary team approach. As the population ages, the number of elderly people with depression will increase and therefore pose an increasing challenge to healthcare services.

Drug therapy

The elderly respond well to pharmacotherapy and all elderly depressed people should be granted the right of adequate treatment with reasonable doses of suitable antidepressants. Over-cautious treatment or failure to treat altogether should be deplored.

The choice of first-line antidepressant will be, to a degree, dictated by the treating clinician's experience and familiarity with the range of antidepressants. In general, outstanding superiority of one class of drug relative to another in terms of effectiveness has not been demonstrated. The choice of antidepressant for a particular patient therefore involves the prescriber in a consideration of the risk/benefit ratio of each treatment. The four key factors to consider are:

- Efficacy
- Tolerability
- Safety
- Potential drug interactions

Efficacy

The first choice should be for a demonstrably effective compound. The conventional tricyclic antidepressants and the newer compounds including the selective serotonin re-uptake inhibitors (SSRIs) are equally effective in treating depression in the elderly.

Tolerability

The elderly are particularly sensitive to drug side-effects and dangerously vulnerable to any consequences of such side-effects. The side-effect profile of the SSRIs renders these compounds more acceptable to many patients and this might be expected to lead to increased compliance. However, the relatively minor side-effects of nausea and anxiety in some patients do reduce compliance.

Safety

Some antidepressants are dangerous if taken in overdose and this must be an important consideration when prescribing to patients who are at risk of suicide or have a history of overdose. The newer compounds are undoubtedly safer in overdose.

Potential drug interactions

Antidepressants, especially the older tricyclic compounds, have a broad pharmacological profile and drug interactions can therefore be a problem. This is especially so in the elderly who, because of multiple pathology, are often prescribed many different classes of drugs. The newer compounds present fewer interaction problems.

When prescribing an antidepressant for the first time a full drug history should be taken. Effective communication between prescribers is essential – the elderly depressed are often treated by different teams such as the primary care

Treatment drug	Interacting drug	Interaction effect
Tricyclic antidepressants	Alcohol and benzodiazepines	Sedation
	Anti-epileptics	Reduced seizure threshold Reduced plasma concentration of some TCAs
	Antihypertensives and diuretics	Hypotension enhanced
	Antipsychotics	Increased antimuscarinic side-effects
	Anti-arrhythmics	Ventricular arrhythmias with TCAs that prolong QT interval
	Antihistamines	Increased antimuscarinic and sedative effects; increased risk of ventricular arrythmias with some antihistamines
	Antimuscarinics	Increased antimuscarinic side-effects
SSRIs*	MAOIs	Increased risk of CNS toxicity (see text and Table 8)
	Sumatriptan	Increased risk of CNS toxicity
	Anti-epileptics	Reduced seizure threshold but plasma concentration of some anti-epileptics increased
	Lithium	Increased risk of CNS toxicity
	Anticoagulants	Effects of warfarin possibly enhanced

*These compounds are chemically distinct and have differing pharmacological profiles which leads to variations in their potential for drug interaction.

For individual drug effects see BNF.

Table 7
Main drug interactions with antidepressants (see British National Formulary Appendix 1 for complete list).

team, an old age psychiatry team and a medicine for the elderly team. In this situation polypharmacy can easily become a problem even with the best of intentions. When changing dosage or class of antidepressants it is good practice to copy a letter highlighting the change to all medical teams involved with the patient.

Where a drug interaction is of possible concern further information can be sought from the British National Formulary, the Data Sheet Compendium or from the local hospital pharmacists. Important interactions with the major antidepressants are listed in Table 7.

Categories of drugs available

Tricyclic antidepressants

These drugs have been in widespread use since the 1960s and there is an enormous body of data on their efficacy and individual side-effect profiles in the elderly. The tricyclics are used as first line treatment by many psychiatrists and are considerably cheaper than newer agents. Because side-effect considerations are the major practical determinant of which tricyclic to use, it is perhaps helpful to consider the major side-effects associated with this class of drugs:

1 All tricyclics have some degree of cardiotoxicity and should not be given to patients with a history of arrhythmias, bundle branch block, abnormal QT interval syndromes or poorly controlled heart failure.

2 Postural hypotension can be an unpleasant and dangerous side-effect in the elderly. Patients taking diuretics and anti-hypertensive treatment are probably at greatest risk and it is good practice to measure lying and standing blood pressure in all patients before considering a tricyclic.

3 Most tricyclics have anticholinergic effects:

Anticholinergic side-effects of tricyclic antidepressants
- Dry mouth
- Confusion
- Blurring of vision
- Worsening of glaucoma
- Urinary retention
- Constipation

---

4 Other side-effects include sedation and fatigue.

Probably the most damaging consequence of these side-effects is upon the confidence of prescribing clinicians who, out of understandable concern, treat patients with inadequate doses of tricyclic. This is probably worse than doing nothing, particularly if it means that the physician does not try an alternative treatment with a more acceptable side-effect profile.

Choice of a particular tricyclic may be made by exploiting, rather than avoiding, side-effects associated with each agent. For example, in a severely agitated patient, a sedative antidepressant such as amitriptyline, mianserin or trazodone may be chosen.

Selective serotonin re-uptake inhibitors (SSRIs)

These drugs have been available for several years and are established as effective, safe and well tolerated by elderly patients. They are as effective as the tricyclics in the treatment of depression. These compounds are chemically distinct and have differing pharmacological profiles which leads to variations in their side-effect profile; prescribing physicians are referred to the datasheets for individual drugs. The side-effects include gastrointestinal problems (including nausea), and tremor, headache, dizziness and sweating for some (but not all) SSRIs. These may be upsetting for the patient, but are often only seen in the first days or weeks on the drug. Compared with the tricyclics, SSRIs lack cardiotoxicity, do not affect the control of blood pressure and do not have anticholinergic activity. Importantly, they appear to be safe in overdose.

Monoamine oxidase inhibitors (MAOIs)

Because of the difficulties involved in avoiding particular foods and combinations of drugs (the elderly are, of course, often on a wide variety of medications) there are practical reasons for avoiding the use of MAOIs in the elderly. They may have a limited place in the treatment of patients with phobic, hypochondriacal or hysterical features.

The sequential treatment of depression with MAOIs and with other antidepressants should be commenced with care and the second drug should only be started after stopping the first and allowing for an appropriate wash-out period (Table 8).

	Wash-out Period
TCA followed by MAOI	1 week
MAOI followed by TCA	2 weeks
Fluoxetine followed by MAOI	5 weeks
Other SSRI followed by MAOI	1–2 weeks
MAOI followed by SSRI	2 weeks

Table 8
Sequential treatment with MAOIs and antidepressants.

Combined treatment of an MAOI and another antidepressant is occasionally used, but only with extreme caution within the hospital setting, and should generally be considered contraindicated.

Lithium

Lithium acts as a mood stabilizer in the prophylaxis of manic depressive psychosis and also has an antidepressant effect. It can be used alone as an antidepressant, or as an adjunct to treatment with a tricyclic antidepressant or SSRI in cases of treatment resistance.

Most elderly patients tolerate lithium well and as long as serum levels are monitored and kept within the range 0.4–0.8 mmol/l, mild degrees of renal impairment, concurrent diuretic therapy and mild heart failure are not contraindications to its use. All patients should have an ECG and baseline urea and electrolytes and thyroid function tests prior to commencing treatment. Thyroid function and urea and electrolytes should be checked at least once every 6 months and a lithium level every 3 months.

In summary

Tricyclic antidepressants are cheap and highly effective but have a side-effect profile (particularly their cardiotoxicity) that can be a major problem in the elderly. The development of SSRIs has been a major advance and the relative safety of this group of compounds has ensured them an important role in drug treatment and a place as first line therapy for many clinicians.

Electroconvulsive therapy

This is a highly effective and safe treatment for depression in elderly patients. In those patients whose lives are at immediate risk through failure to eat and drink, suicidal behaviour or severe retardation it is the treatment of choice. The risks involved in having ECT are essentially those associated with any brief general anaesthetic. Although some anaesthetists may be anxious about giving a general anaesthetic to patients within 3 months of a myocardial infarction or stroke, the only real absolute contraindication to ECT is the clinical evidence of raised intracranial pressure. Medically frail patients are generally far more at risk from their depression if it is untreated than they are from ECT.

Most hospitals give ECT twice weekly to inpatients. Confusion only very unusually persists for more than an hour or so after each treatment. If persistent confusion is a problem, unilateral ECT may be given or the treatments given only once per week. Treatment should continue until mood has improved, typically after five to ten applications. Patients should be established on a maintenance antidepressant (either a tricyclic or an SSRI) during ECT treatment, otherwise they are in danger of relapse on cessation of the ECT.

ECT can be given to patients who refuse it, or who are incapable of giving consent for it, if they are detained on a treatment Section (such as Section 3) of the Mental Health Act, and a doctor appointed by the Mental Health Act Commission provides a second opinion which confirms that the treatment is necessary.

Treatment-resistant depression

A small proportion of patients with depression will not recover, despite four to six weeks of treatment with adequate antidepressant doses. In such cases, treatment with either ECT or augmentation of drug treatment with lithium or another class of antidepressant (e.g. adding an SSRI to existing treatment with a tricyclic) is often effective (Fig. 8).

Psychotic depression

Associated psychotic features are particularly common in the depressed elderly and can take the form of distressing nihilistic and hypochondriacal delusions or tormenting hallucinations. Although some psychiatrists routinely prescribe antipsychotic medication for such patients, it is important to remember that the psychotic symptoms arise out of a depressed mood, and so the best treatment for them is one that improves mood quickly, and this means ECT.

Prophylaxis

Studies in the elderly have demonstrated an unequivocal benefit of long term treatment to prevent relapse of depression. Treatment after a first episode should continue for at least 4–6 months after symptomatic recovery and some studies indicate up to 2 years.

Many psychiatrists believe that the prophylaxis of a relapsing and serious condition such as depression is an indication for life long treatment. However, patients should not stay on anti-depressants without regular review. At review, serious consideration should be given to the appropriate time to stop prescribing. This might be after two years of remission, the development of side-effects, the onset of physical illness or with increasing frailty.

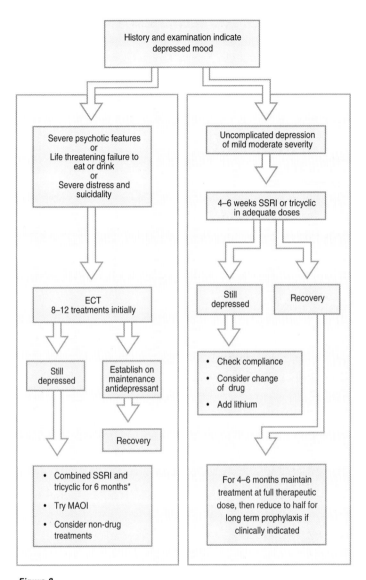

Figure 8
Treatment algorithm for depression in the elderly.
* *Because of interaction problems this should only be undertaken in a hospital setting by a psychiatric team.*

There is evidence that concomitant psychotherapy and involvement in outpatient groups where psychological treatments are offered may also act as effective prophylaxis against relapse of depression.

Psychological treatments for depression

Psychotherapy

Psychotherapy should not be ignored as a treatment option in the elderly and there is a growing interest in this field. Individual or group psychotherapy is most effective in the treatment of depression in elderly patients if combined with antidepressant therapy. The goals of therapy should be explicit, although therapists should not be too pessimistic about the capacity for change in elderly individuals. Studies have indicated that both the psychodynamic and cognitive-behavioural approaches are equally successful with the elderly, although the mechanisms of the effect of psychotherapy are not understood, and it is probably more important to match a therapist and a patient with a therapeutic model that both find acceptable. Some authors have suggested that the life review approach, in which patients are encouraged to achieve a resolution of the life cycle as a positive experience, may not be effective in the treatment of depressed patients who may see their lives in a very negative light.

Cognitive therapy

As the only psychological treatment designed specifically for depression and with its directed, focused and time-limited nature, cognitive therapy seems a particularly appropriate method for treating older depressed patients. Studies have investigated the use of cognitive therapy with medically ill patients and shown some improvements in functioning and mental state when the therapy is given by physicians.

Cognitive therapy is built upon a model of depression that proposes a cognitive triad that develops in a depressed individual. The individual acquires a negative view of self, their future and the world. They believe, to varying degrees, that they are useless or inadequate, that their future is unrelentingly bleak and hopeless and that the outside world or their experiences are deprived, obstructive or diminished. The cognitive model of depression accounts for the development of this negative triad by postulating that the depression-prone individual has underlying negative schemata. These are personal models of how we make sense of events and are relatively stable throughout life. An individual prone to developing depression has a predominantly negative set of schemata and interprets positive or neutral events in a negative light. These negative schemata lead to a typically depressive set of thinking patterns that lead the patient to take events out of context or to overgeneralize. A home-help failing to attend is interpreted as an act of personal dislike for the patient; a daughter failing to telephone is taken as evidence by the elderly depressed patient that they are unwanted, unloved and a burden to all the family.

This model provides a context within which to understand the patient and can be helpful as a tool to aid recovery. While research evidence for the veracity of the model is somewhat lacking, the model has provided one of the most important advances in our understanding of the non-biological processes involved in depression and has proved of some use to a wide range of professionals.

The cognitive-behavioural therapy based upon this model aims to inform the patient of their thought processes and help correct the negative aspects of these. The model is explained to the patient and studies have demonstrated that the elderly are receptive to this type of understanding, although explanation should be brief and focused. The link between thoughts and moods is then demonstrated to the patient using their own experiences. It can help if the patient keeps a diary of their mood and actions between appointments. Through specific exercises, activity schedules and graded task assignments, cognitive therapy aims to modify behaviour and mode of thinking. Negative thoughts are identified and challenged in the therapy session itself.

As an example, an elderly woman with depression may complain that she was ignored by the staff at a day centre. Questioning might identify the negative thought that this perceived slighting was interpreted by the patient as evidence that she was disliked and therefore worthless. This could be challenged by encouraging the patient to identify other reasons why she might have been ignored. The realization that the day centre workers were particularly busy because of staff sickness might go some way to alleviating the distress. Exercises to counter negative thinking can be given – in this case the elderly patient might be encouraged to be pro-active and approach the staff herself. Review of the 'homework' exercises at the following session might demonstrate that the staff responded well to the approach and the original negative thought was dispelled.

Therapy is never as simple as this trivial example but studies have demonstrated that the elderly do have this dysfunctional form of thinking in depression and that this can be corrected. Studies have shown that over a relatively short period of therapy the depressed can be taught to identify and counter negative thoughts and that this does result in some therapeutic benefit. Unfortunately, there are few studies of the efficacy of cognitive therapy in the treatment of depression in the elderly, although those that have been conducted show a therapeutic benefit similar to that seen in the younger population. In one respect the elderly depressed have an advantage over young people with depression, in that they have a lifetime of experience with which to counter negative thoughts associated with a current depressive episode.

Anxiety management

Since depressive illness in the elderly is frequently complicated by anxiety symptoms which may not resolve when mood has been successfully treated, referral for anxiety management is often necessary. Techniques used most commonly include progressive relaxation programmes, either alone with a pre-recorded tape or in a group supervised by a psychologist or occupational therapist. Anxiety management is successful in a proportion of the elderly and need not be restricted to a service provided by hospital-based units. General practice-based counsellors or therapists have an important role in providing these treatments. In our experience however, the elderly benefit from treatment together and do not always fit in well with anxiety management groups comprising patients of all ages.

Family therapy

Family problems may contribute to the development of a depressive illness, and the support of a patient's family is most important in ensuring a successful outcome to treatment. Family dynamics change with ageing of the family unit and the aged family member moves from a position of dominance to a position of some dependence. This can invoke a variety of feelings in the younger members of the family ranging from pity to anger and sometimes feelings of sadism which may, obviously, be difficult to admit. Most of those who treat the elderly recognize that adult children can have a wide range of feelings towards their elderly, depressed and dependant parent, and that at times these feelings can perpetuate the depressive episode or at least hinder recovery. The aims of family therapy with the relatives of depressed patients are to relieve some of the feelings of frustration and despair that the illness may have provoked in them, and to remove attitudes and structures within the family that may be detrimental to recovery. Family therapy is usually given by trained therapists in hospital-based departments. Increasingly, old age psychiatrists are gaining experience in this field and all, even if not giving family therapy themselves, can usefully gain from the insights that this field has to offer.

The role of the multidisciplinary team

Most elderly patients with depression will be assessed and treated by their general practitioner alone, without recourse to psychiatric or community nursing services. However, not only the most severely ill or treatment-resistant patients benefit from specialist input and most local old age psychiatry services would very much welcome referral of depressed individuals from general practitioners early in the course of the illness. Following referral, members of the multidisciplinary team, including the general practitioner, may be involved at any of several stages.

Assessment

Most elderly patients with depression can be assessed and treated by a general practitioner without referral to an old age psychiatry multi-disciplinary team. However, in cases of uncertain diagnosis, for moderate or for severe depressive episodes and in cases with multiple social and physical problems, referral to secondary services should always be considered. In some services the initial assessment will be performed by a non-medical member of the team and in all services a multi-disciplinary approach is now the norm.

An initial assessment may be carried out in the patient's home, at the general practice surgery if a local psychiatrist carries out regular clinics there, or in the outpatient department of the hospital. At this point, the psychiatrist and general practitioner will be involved in assessing the severity of depression, exploring possible aetiological and precipitating factors and reviewing the effects of previously applied treatments. Assessments of support networks and of suicidal risk can also be made at this time.

Treatment

Once the local old age psychiatry team has become involved, they can advise on the most appropriate treatment and help to decide whether the patient should be admitted or can be treated as an outpatient or day patient.

The occupational therapist in many cases is instrumental in assessing the home environment and ensuring adaptations to maintain maximal function in the physically disabled or the frail. Often this intervention is a major contributor to recovery from depression. Occupational therapy is the most important component of the day hospital care, and interventions range from increasing physical exercise and mobility through structured activities to therapeutic groups. The occupational therapist might also have an important input into the day-to-day care of depressed patients attending social services' day centres or those in residential settings. The psychologist on the team has an important role in undertaking cognitive or behavioural therapies if these are indicated, and may also offer indispensable insights into psychosocial factors related to aetiology. In patients presenting a diagnostic problem between dementia and depression or where there is an admixture of the two, detailed psychometric testing often resolves the issue and in any case provides baseline measures for future reference.

Allocation of a community psychiatric nurse is important, particularly in the early stages of treatment when the patient may be difficult for the family to manage without support, and to monitor for medication side-effects or non-compliance. Obviously there is more to the treatment of depression than the prescribing of antidepressant medication and the skills of other members of the team such as occupational therapists and psychologists can be exploited during this time.

Maintaining recovery and monitoring for relapse

Once a patient has been successfully treated and their mood has improved, everything that can be done to prevent relapse should be provided. Long-term follow-up by a community psychiatric nurse or continued attendance at the day hospital may be as important for prophylaxis as the continued prescription of antidepressants. Resources under the control of local social services, such as day centres, home helps and workers from voluntary agencies like Age Concern can all be recruited.

The partner of the depressed patient should not be forgotten both as an important part of the process to maintain recovery and as a person vulnerable to depression in their own right. The community psychiatric nurse or day hospital team should take time to assess the needs of carers and notify the general practitioner if there are particular concerns. A carer-spouse might be directed to a carers group either within the hospital setting or attached to a general practitioner's surgery. Other groups are run by voluntary and charitable organizations.

Prevention of depression in the elderly

No effective strategies have yet been reliably determined for preventing depression in the elderly. However, clinical depression is almost certainly on a spectrum of mood that ranges from mild unhappiness and misery to major depressive disorder. It is not known whether those with sub-clinical depressed mood progress to clinical depressive disorder but this does seem possible. The old age psychiatry multi-disciplinary team might have a role to play in preventing depression in the elderly. It is possible that by providing input into residential and nursing homes, by initiating or running carers groups, or by encouraging an interest in the isolated elderly within social services departments, some individuals can be prevented from suffering from depression. There has been something of a progression within the field of old age psychiatry; first the identification of depression in the elderly population was improved; now the task is to ensure adequate treatment for all patients; perhaps the task for the future is to contribute towards the prevention of depression in individuals as they reach the latter part of their lives.

Bibliography

Abas MA, Sahakian BJ and Levy R (1990) Neuropsychological deficits and CT scan changes in elderly depressives. *Psychological Medicine* **20**: 507–520.

Ames D, Ashby D, Mann AH and Graham N (1988) Psychiatric illness in elderly residents of Part III homes in one London borough: prognosis and review. *Age and Ageing* **17**: 249–256.

Baldwin R (1988) Delusional and non-delusional depression in late life: evidence for distinct subtypes. *British Journal of Psychiatry* **152**: 39–44.

Baldwin RC and Jolley DJ (1986) Prognosis of depression in old age. *British Journal of Psychiatry* **149**: 574–583.

Benbow SB (1989) The role of electroconvulsive therapy in the treatment of depressive illness in old age. *British Journal of Psychiatry* **155**: 147–152.

Blazer DG, Batchar JR and Manton K (1986) Suicide in late life. *Journal of the American Geriatric Society* **34**: 519–525.

Copeland JRM, Dewey ME, Wood N, Searle R, Davidson IA and McWilliam C (1987) Range of mental illness among the elderly in the community: prevalence in Liverpool using the GMS-AGECAT package. *British Journal of Psychiatry* **150**: 815–823.

Corcoran E, Guerandel A and Wrigley M (1994) The day hospital in the psychiatry of old age – what difference does it make? *Irish Journal of Psychological Medicine* **11**: 110–115.

Godber C, Rosenvinge H, Wilkinson D and Smithies J (1987). Depression in old age. Prognosis after ECT. *International Journal of Geriatric Psychiatry* **2**: 19–24.

Gottfries CG and Nyth AL (1991) Effect of citalopram, a selective 5HT reuptake blocker, in emotionally disturbed patients with dementia. *Annals of New York Academy of Science* **640**: 276–279.

Gottfries CG, Karlsson I and Nyth AL (1992). Treatment of depression in elderly patients with and without dementia disorders. *International Clinical Psychopharmacology* **6** (Supplement: 5) 55–64.

Jacoby RJ, Dolan RJ, Levy R and Baldy R (1983) Quantitative computed tomography in elderly depressed patients. *British Journal of Psychiatry* **143**: 124–127.

Katona CLE (1994) *Depression in Old Age* (Chichester: John Wiley & Sons).

Macdonald AJD (1986) Do general practitioners miss depression in elderly patients? *British Medical Journal* **292**: 1365–1367.

Murphy E (1982) Social origins of depression in old age. *British Journal of Psychiatry* **141**: 135–142.

Murphy E and Brown GW (1980) Life events, psychiatric disturbance and physical illness. *British Journal of Psychiatry* **136**: 326–328.

NIH Consensus Development Panel (1992) Diagnosis and treatment of depression in late life. *Journal of the American Medical Association* **268**: 1018–1024.

Nyth AL, Gottfries CG, Lyby K, Smedegaard-Anderson L et al (1992) A controlled multi-centre clinical study of citalopram and placebo in elderly depressed patients with and without concomitant dementia. *Acta Psychiatria Scandinavica* **86**: 138–145.

Old Age Depression Interest Group (1993) How long should the elderly take antidepressants? A double-blind placebo-controlled study of continuation prophylaxis therapy with dothiepin. *British Journal of Psychiatry* **162**: 175–182.

Salzman C, Schneider LS, Lebowitz BD (1993) Antidepressant treatment of very old patients. *American Journal of Geriatric Psychiatry* **1**: 21–29.

Yesavage JA, Brink TL, Rose TL, Lum O (1983) Development and validation of a geriatric depression screening scale: a preliminary report. *Journal of Psychiatric Research* **17**: 37–49.

Index

Page numbers in *italic* refer to the illustrations

V

W

X